This book is dedicated to anyone who has ever suffered from debilitating stress.

May this sequence help those who continue to fight through the heaviness of stress.

The Vagus Nerve is the longest cranial nerve in the body. It starts at the base of the skull and extends all the way down to the heart, lungs, digestive tract, and other abdominal organs. It controls our fight or flight response. People with low vagal tone may frequently suffer from sickness, negative moods, depression, and heart issues. People with optimal vagal tone are more resilient under stress and healthier.

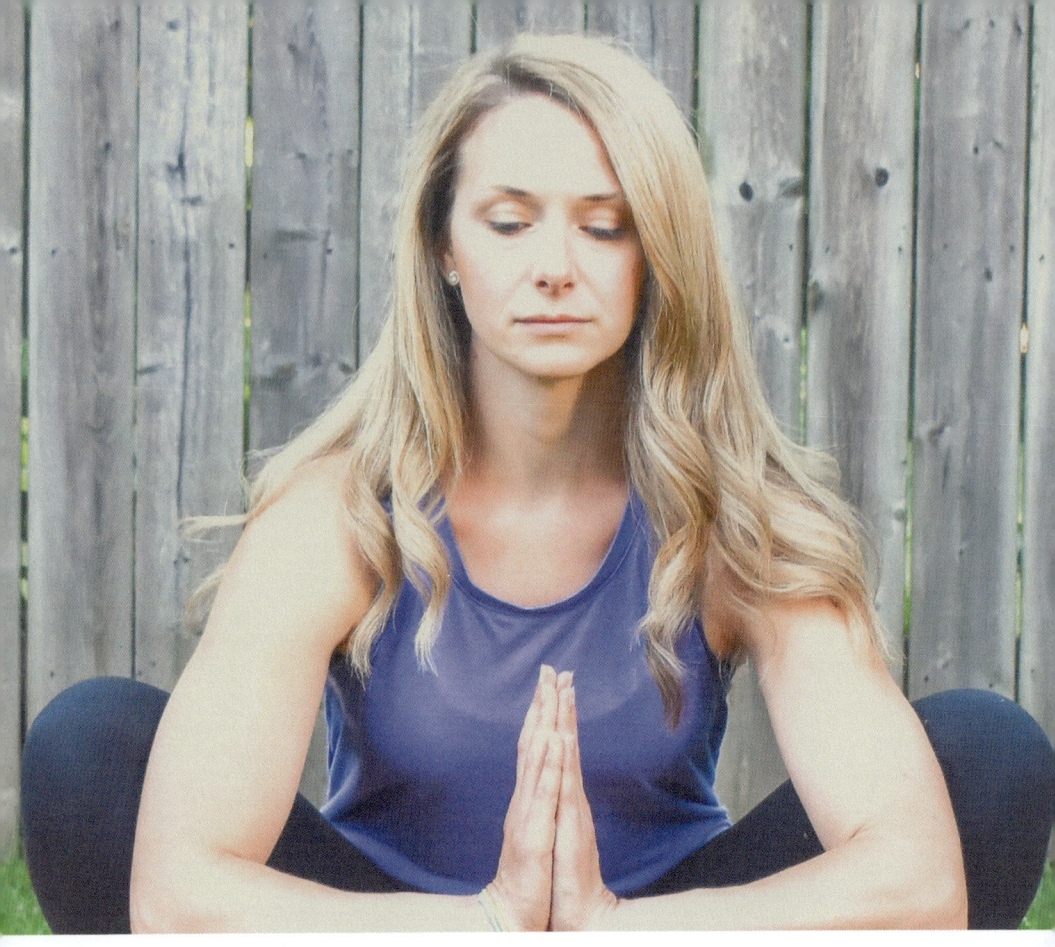

Centering

Begin on your back. Place one hand on your stomach and your other hand on your heart.

Notice your breath. It's already there, you don't have to search for it. Just notice it. Notice what it feels like as the air enters your nose. Notice what it feels like to hold it for a second and let it out.

Feel the firmness of the floor under you. It's able to hold you. Let your bones sink into it.

Bring your attention to your forehead, your eyes, your nose. Squeeze your eyes shut, letting your forehead and nose also scrunch up. Release.

Bring your attention to your jaw. Clench your teeth. Release. Pull your tongue away from the roof of your mouth.

Bring your attention to your shoulders. Pull them to your ears, squeezing the muscles. Release, pulling them back down away from the ears. Let your shoulder blades slide down your back.

Bring your attention to your hands. Make them into tight fists. Release.

Bring your attention to your thighs and your knees. Tighten those muscles, squeezing your legs together. Release.

Bring your attention to your feet. Squeeze your toes together, engage those muscles. Release, letting your feet just fall to the sides.

Take three breaths here, feeling each one move in through your nostrils and back out.

Bring both knees to your chest and hug them in tight. Take two breaths.

Place your right hand on your left knee and bring both knees to your right side. Extend your left arm out to the side, or bend it like a cactus. Turn your head to your left. Hold here for 3 breaths.

Hug your knees back into the center. Repeat twist for the other side. Hold for three breaths.

The Vagus Nerve is also called the Wandering Nerve since it travels through so much of our body and has an impact on nearly every function. In a way, we are also wanderers. You move through your day leaving pieces of yourself everywhere. There's a part of you still at work, wondering if you've missed anything that needed to be done. There's a part of you still at the store, wondering if you were too short with the check out guy because you were in a rush and things were not moving at your speed. There's a part of you still at home, checking off all the things that need doing; or still having a tense conversation with your significant other and coming up with better responses to the rude thing they said to you. Leave all of those places. Bring yourself back to you.

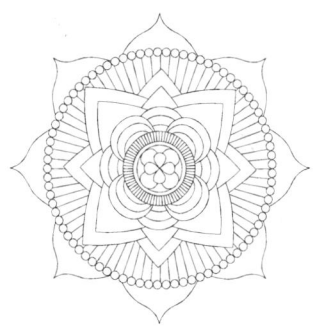

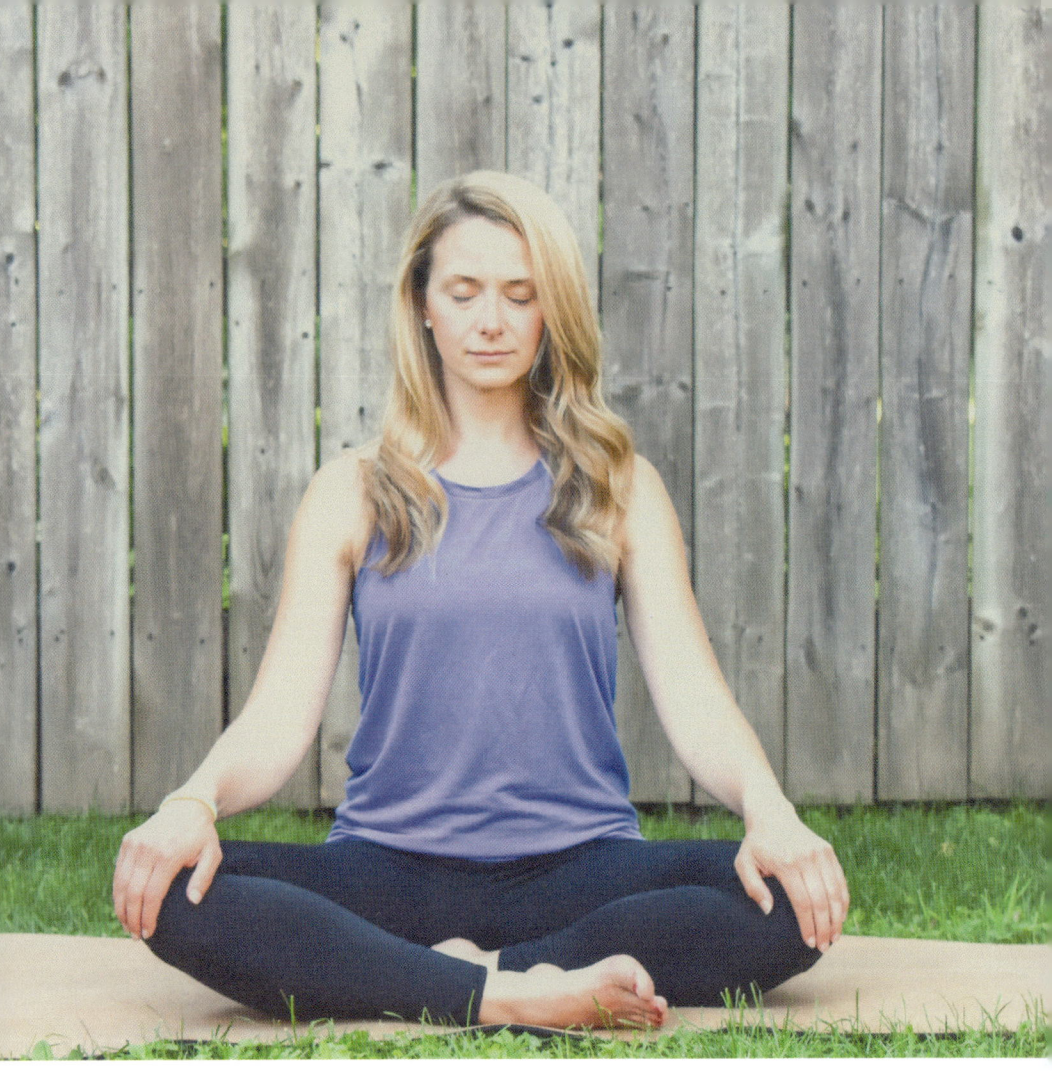

Bandhas

Roll to your side and come up to a seated position with your legs crossed. Make sure you're comfortable.

*It can feel more comfortable sometimes if you sit on something, like a block or bolster or a rolled blanket. This brings your hips higher than your knees and allows your legs to relax a little more.

One way to draw ourselves back in from where we are wandering is to use locks. Locks can help us contain our energy.

For the first lock, engage the floor muscles of the pelvis. This is the root lock and it tones your pelvic floor and provides more support to your lower back. So draw your attention down into your pelvic floor and engage those deep muscles, drawing them up to your navel. Release.

Do this one more time. Release.

For the second lock, place your hands on your sides, like you are holding your ribs. There are muscles here: your transverse abdominals. Use these muscles to draw everything between your hands up and into your rib cage. Don't force or squeeze. These locks should be gentle. It's like giving yourself internal hugs. Release.

Draw everything in one more time. Release.

Extend your legs long and remove any props you may be using.

Myelin is a fatty, white substance that wraps around the end of many nerve cells. It forms an electrically insulating sheath that increases nerve condition speeds. Myelin is critical for optimal brain function and mental health.

It allows your brain to send information faster and more efficiently, making it essential for the optimal functioning of your nervous system. Demyelination can happen when the myelin that insulates your nerves is destroyed or deteriorates, leading to mental health symptoms and neurodegenerative diseases.

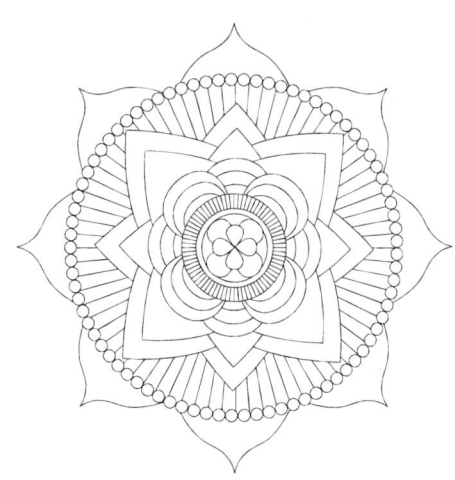

Warm Up

Draw your right knee in and hug it to your chest. Bring your right leg over your left and place your left hand on your knee or outside of your right leg. Place your right hand behind your on the floor and on your next exhale turn your ribcage to the right for a twist. Hold here for three breaths. Repeat on the other side.

Come onto your hands and knees, keeping your back flat, in table position.

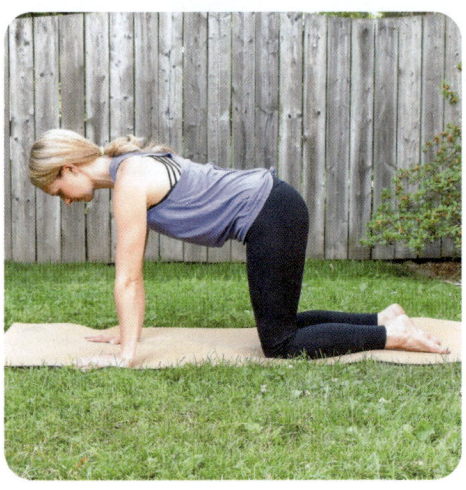

Move through cat and cow poses: on the exhale drop your chin to your chest, pull your navel to your spine, draw your tailbone and sit bones down. Arch your back like a cat, pulling your shoulder blades apart

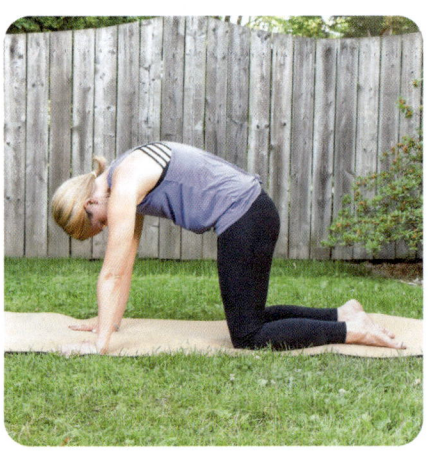

Then on the inhale, slowly drop your navel back down, lifting your chin, sit bones, and sternum, like a cow.

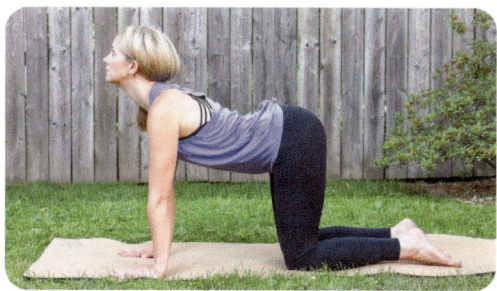

Do this four times.

Come back to table position. Keep your knees under your hips and your hands under your shoulders.

Engage your locks. This will help with balance for the next moves.

Lift your right knee and let it hover, then bring it up into a lateral leg lift. Bring it back to a hover. Do this two more times.

Repeat for the left leg.

Draw your right knee toward your forehead, and your forehead toward your knee. Then press your heel all the way back, extending your leg behind you. Make sure your hip points are both even and pointing down. Lift your left arm in front of you. Hold here for one breath. Bring both legs and arm down.

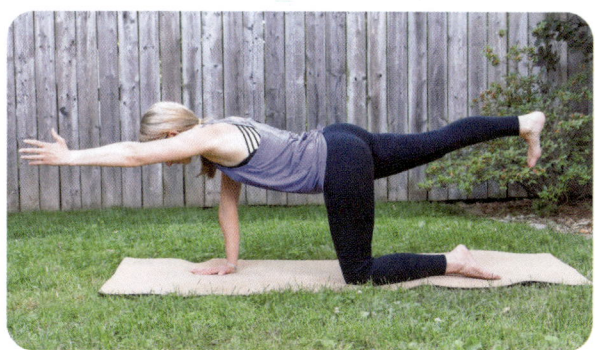

Repeat on the other side.

*By strengthening the Vagus Nerve, researchers are discovering that many conditions can potentially be treated, including Alzheimer's, MS, headaches, depression, and pain. Working to strengthen the Vagus Nerve reduces inflammation, and can contribute to the regeneration of myelin in the brain. All of the movements and poses in this sequence work to strengthen the Vagus Nerve.

Positions

Curl your toes under and push yourself into downward dog. Lift your sit bones, keep your knees bent a little, let your head hang. Keep your heels lifted. Your weight should be evenly distributed between your hands and feet. Shift around, stretching your legs by putting one heel down, then the other. Take five breaths here.

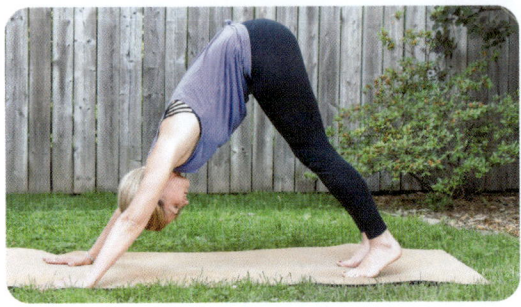

Walk your hands back to your feet and let your head, arms, and torso hang in forward fold. Knees can be bent. Lift partway to a flat back, placing your hands on your shins, then let yourself fall back down again into forward fold.

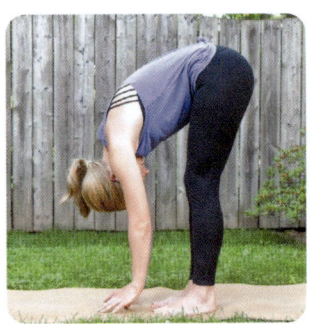 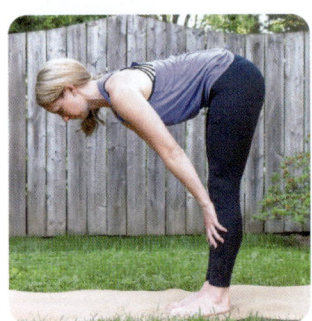

On the inhale, lift yourself all the way up, bringing arms above your head. On the exhale, dive back down. Do this slowly, three more times.

While still in forward fold, ground your feet into the floor. Bend your knees and lift your arms over your as you bring your torso up into chair position. Engage your locks. Hold for three breaths.

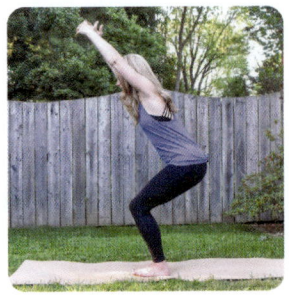

Fold your torso back over your thighs and place hands on the floor. Press fingers into the ground and step left leg back into low lunge. Bring arms overhead. Take five breaths.

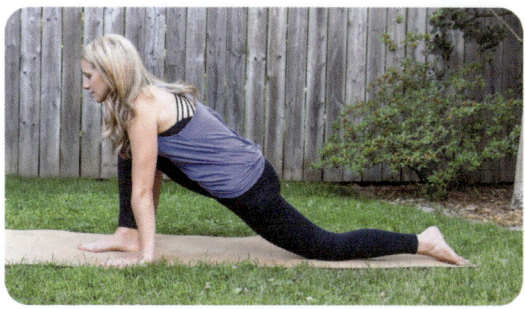

Bring arms in front, pressing palms together. Inhale and lift your chest, exhale and twist toward your front leg.

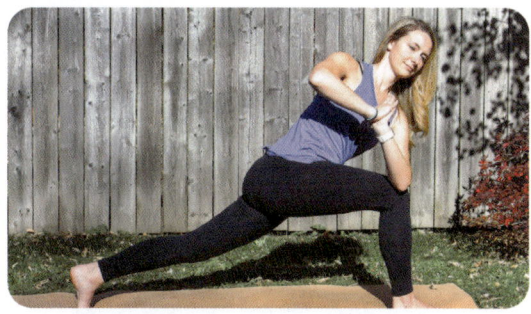

Open arms and place your left hand into the ground on the inside of the front foot. Lift your right arm towards the ceiling.

Begin to shift your weight to your front leg, drawing your back leg in until you can lift it into a twisted half moon. Engage your locks. Press your lifted heel back. *You may find that using a block or something similar helps with stability. Keep your toes on the mat if lifting your leg is too challenging at this time

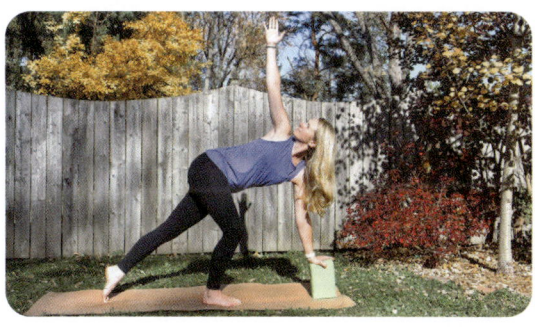

Slowly bring your right hand down to the floor while keeping your left leg lifted behind you. Roll your left hip so that your torso now faces the left, and lift your left arm to the ceiling. You are now in half moon.

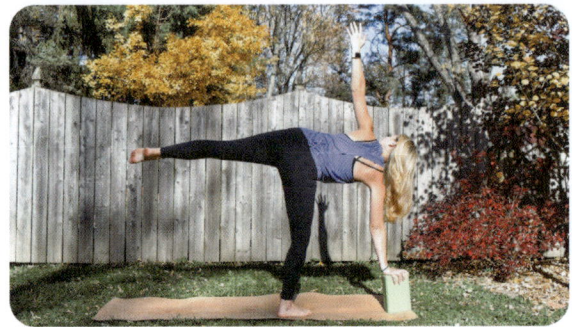

Step your left leg down slowly into warrior 2, keeping your front knee bent. Extend your arms out.

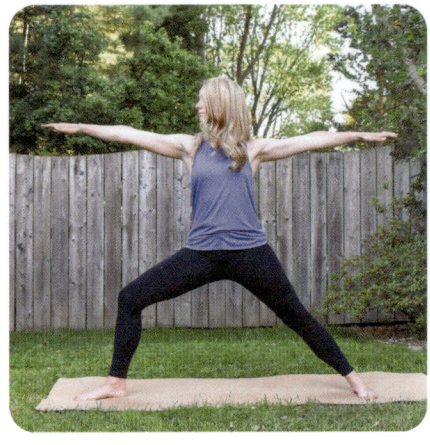

Bring your right arm to your right thigh, lifting your left arm over your head.

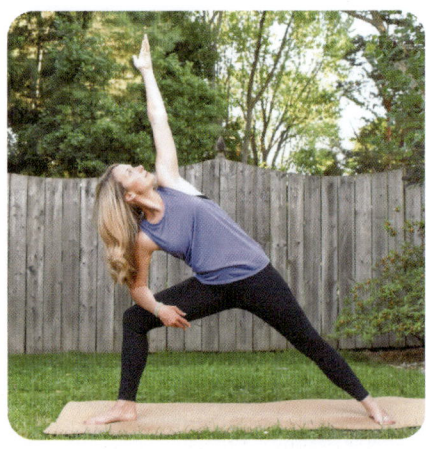

Now slide your left arm down your back leg, lifting your right arm over your head as you lean back into peaceful warrior.

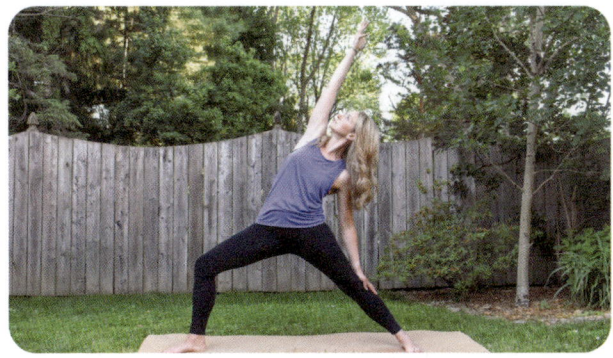

Do this four more times.

Turn your right foot so that it is parallel with your left. Your feet are still wide apart. Place your hand on your hip points and fold forward into a wide-legged forward fold. Let your arms and head hang.

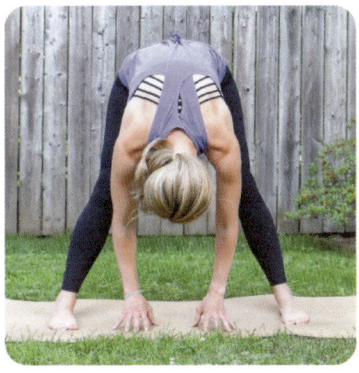

Turn your feet so your toes are pointing out and place your hands back on your hip points. Lift your torso slowly. Once upright, sink your hips, bending your knees into Goddess pose. Engage your locks.

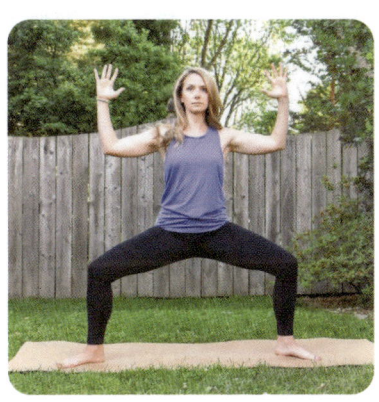

Bring your arms in front of you, placing your left arm over your right into eagle. Fold forward again. Take three breaths.

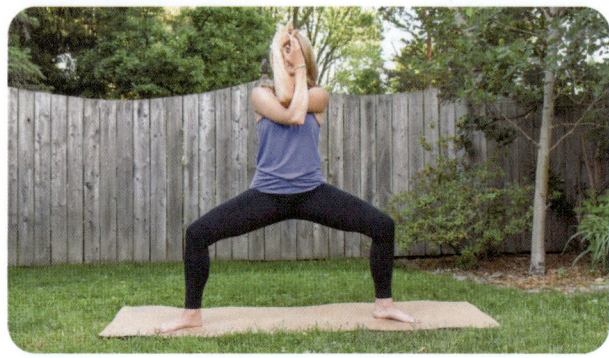

Come up and unwind your arms. Turn right toes back to the front of the mat and place both hands down on either side of your right foot, into low lunge.

Lift right foot back to meet the left, in plank.

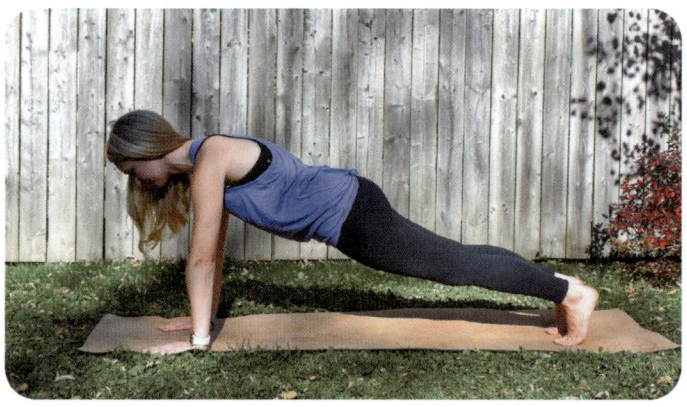

Sink back into child's pose. Take five breaths.

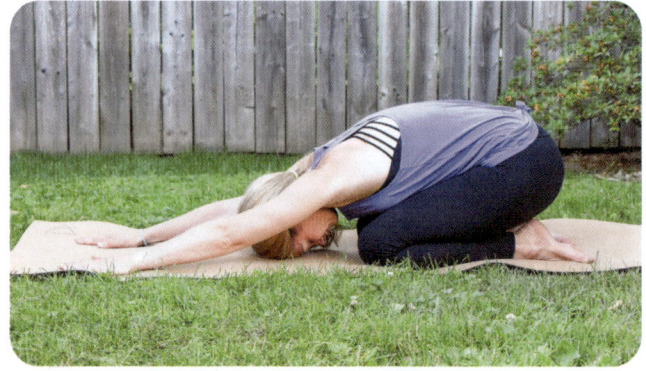

Other Side

Curl your toes under and push yourself into downward dog. Lift your sit bones, keep your knees bent a little, let your head hang. Keep your heels lifted. Take five breaths here.

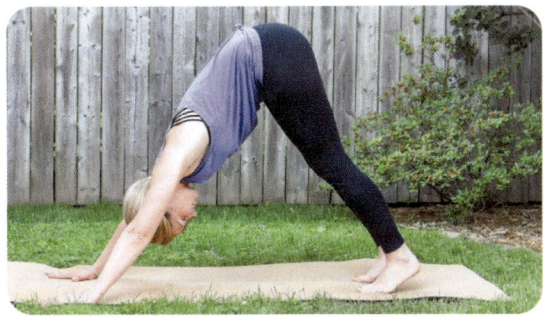

Step forward so your feet meet your hands and let your head, arms, and torso hang in forward fold. Knees can be bent. Lift partway to a flat back, placing your hands on your shins, then let yourself fall back down again into forward fold.

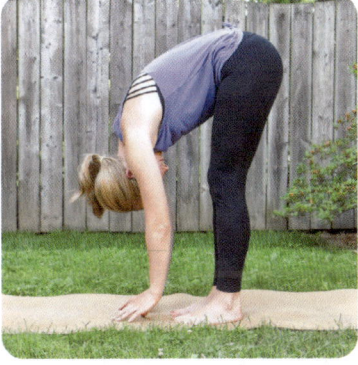

On the inhale, lift yourself all the way up, bringing arms above your head. On the exhale dive back down. Do this slowly, three more times.

While still in forward fold, ground your feet into the floor. Bend your knees and lift your arms over your head as you bring your torso up into chair position. Engage your locks. Hold for three breaths.

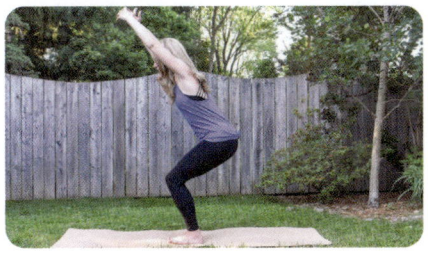

Fold your torso back over your thighs and place hands on the floor. Press fingers into the ground and step right leg back into low lunge. Bring arms overhead. Take five breaths.

Bring arms in front, pressing palms together. Inhale and lift your chest, exhale and twist toward your front leg.

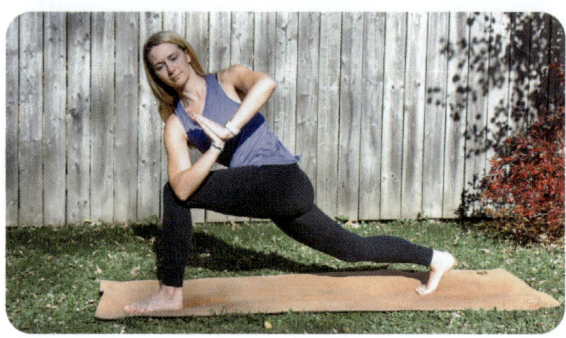

Open arms and place your right hand into the ground on the inside of the front foot. Lift left arm towards the ceiling.

Begin to shift your weight to your front leg, drawing your back leg in until you can lift it into a twisted half moon. Engage your locks. Press your lifted heel back.

Slowly bring your left hand down to the floor while keeping your right leg lifted behind you. Roll your right hip so that your torso now faces the right, and lift your right arm to the ceiling. You are now in half moon.

Step your right leg down slowly into warrior two, keeping your front knee bent. Extend your arms out.

Bring your left arm to your left thigh, lifting your right arm over your head. Now slide your right arm down your back leg, lifting your left arm over your head as you lean back into peaceful warrior. Do this four more times.

Turn your left foot so that it is parallel with your right. Your feet are still wide apart. Place your hands on your hip points and fold forward into a wide-legged forward fold. Let your arms and head hang.

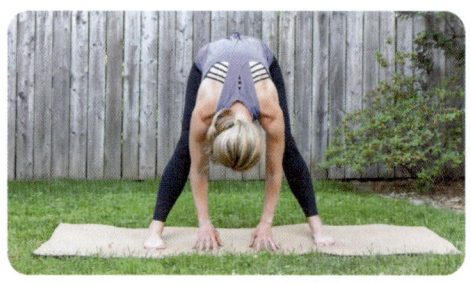

Turn your feet so your toes are pointing out and place your hands back on your hip points. Lift your torso slowly. Once upright, sink your hips, bending your knees into Goddess pose. Engage your locks.

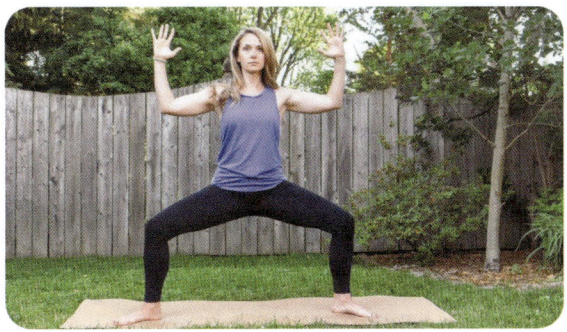

Bring your arms in front of you, placing your right arm over your left into eagle. Fold forward again. Take three breaths.

Come up and unwind your arms. Turn left toes back to the front of the mat and place both hands down on either side of your left foot, into low lunge.

Lift left foot back to meet the right, in plank.

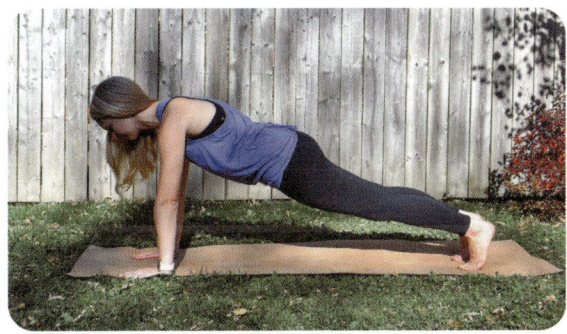

Sink back into child's pose. Take five breaths.

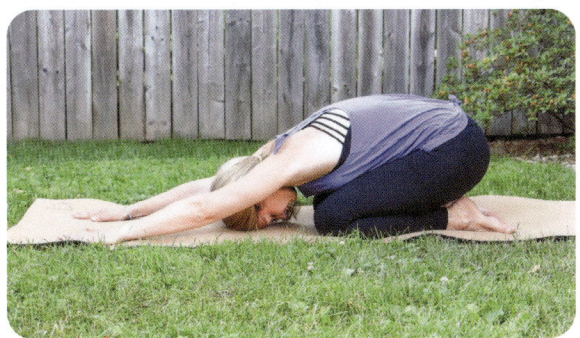

Cool Down

Come into a seated position. Legs crossed in from of you. Intertwine your fingers and place your hands behind your head, cupping your occipital bones.

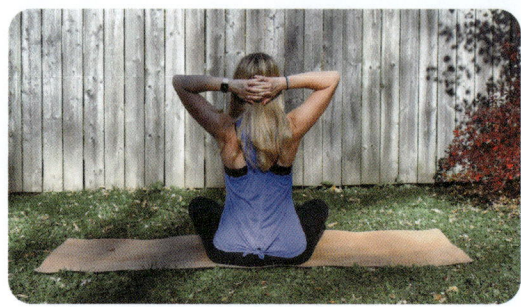

Do the Vagus Nerve release exercise: keeping your head still, look with your eyes about 45 degrees to your left. Blinking is ok, and make sure you keep breathing. When you feel yourself sigh, yawn, or swallow, bring your eyes back to the front. Repeat on the other side.

Come onto your back. Place your hands under your sacrum (lower back) with your palms on the floor. Lift your legs straight up to the ceiling. Hold here and take 10 breaths.

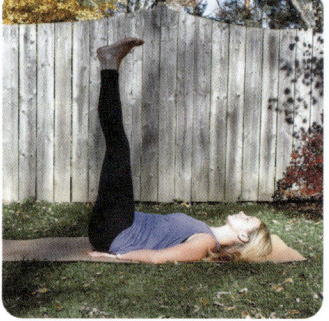

Bring your legs down, and place a bolster, block, or rolled blanket behind you. If it's a bolster or blanket, it should be longways, under your spine. If a block, place it just below your shoulder blades. Lay back in a supported fish pose. Stay here for a few minutes, feeling your chest open.

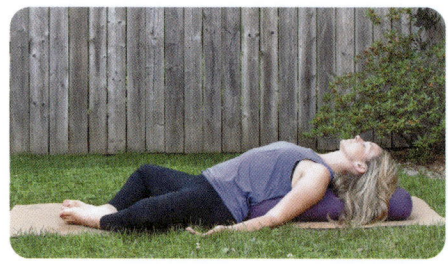

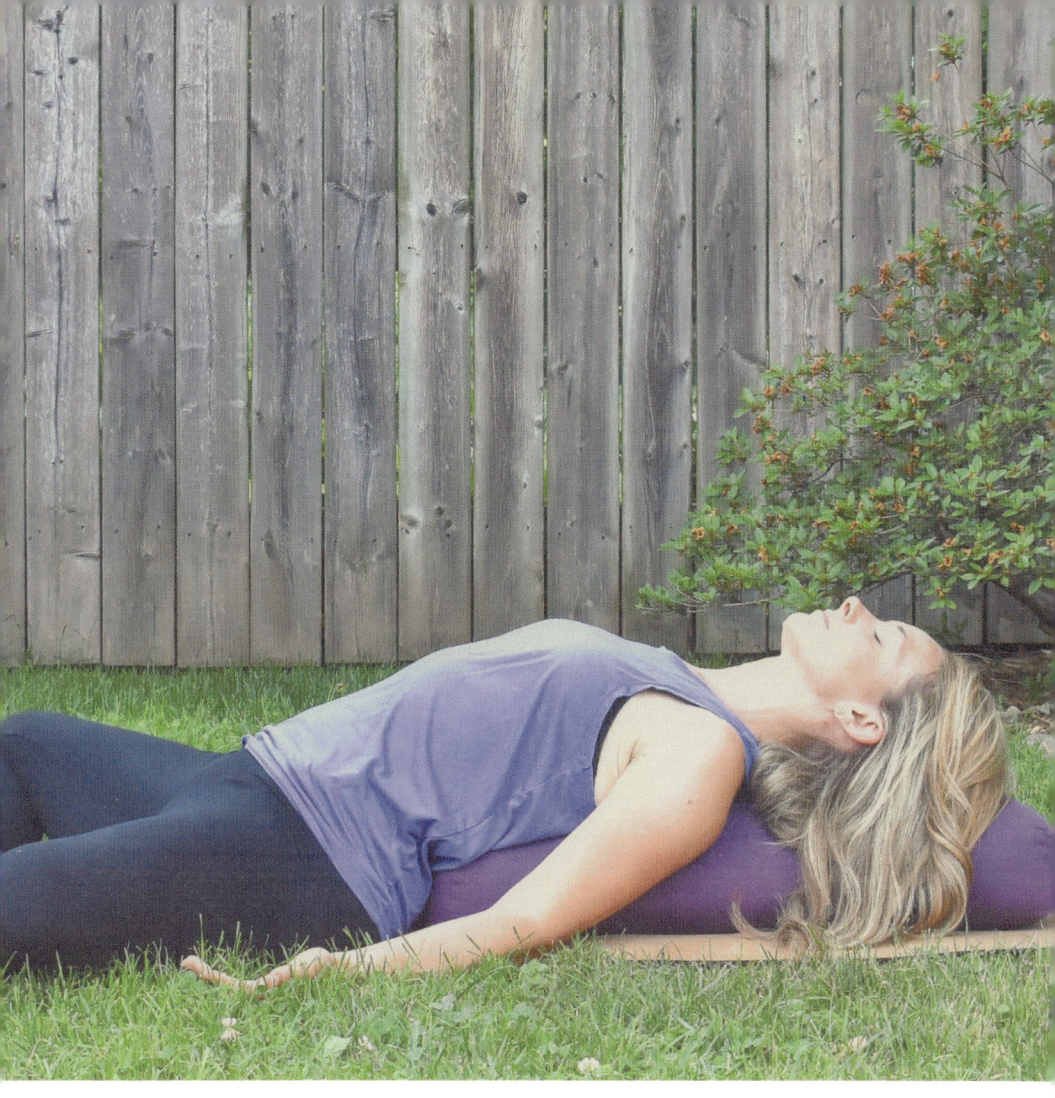

Savasana

Remove any props and lay flat on your back, palms up. Close your eyes. Feel your breath again, and notice any differences in your body. Stay here for a few minutes.

*You are whole just as you are. You do not require anything or anyone else to complete you or make you into you. You are everything you need. Whenever you feel as though you are leaving pieces of yourself around, know that you have the ability to bring yourself back together.

Printed in Great Britain
by Amazon